Fauci

The Bernie Madoff of Science and the HIV
Ponzi Scheme that Concealed the Chronic
Fatigue Syndrome Epidemic

Charles Ortleb

Introduction

This little book consists of a chapter about Anthony Fauci from *The Chronic Fatigue Epidemic Cover-up Volume Two*. It includes a new afterword.

*

If justice and truth prevail in the world, one day what has been called "AIDS" will be renamed "Holocaust II." While gay people were secondary victims of what is referred to as "The Holocaust," or "Holocaust I," they were the main attraction in "Holocaust II." The heterosexist motivation of their stigmatization and persecution in both holocausts were similar even if the manner in which they were harmed was different. I have used the term "Iatrogenocide" to describe what happened to gay men (and others) during Holocaust II.

I was a witness to the AIDS epidemic from the very beginning. As the publisher and editor-in-chief of *New York Native,* I inadvertently oversaw the reporting of the very first story about the epidemic. After hearing about a strange pneumonia occurring in gay men in New York City, I asked a physician to make inquiries with the public health authorities. In a story headlined "Disease Rumors Largely Unfounded" published in our May 18, 1981 issue, Dr. Lawrence Mass wrote, "Last week there were rumors that an exotic new disease had hit the gay community in New York. Here are the facts. From the New York City Department of Health, Dr. Steve Phillips explained that the rumors are for the most part unfounded. Each year, approximately 12 to 24 cases of infection with a protozoa-like organism, Pneumocystis carinii, are reported in New York City area. The organism is not exotic; in fact, it's ubiquitous. But most of us have a natural or easily acquired immunity."

Six weeks later it turned out that the rumors were true when the CDC reported on the first cases of what would be called AIDS. It is hard to overstate the shock and terror that gripped the gay community in New York City and eventually around the world. People dreaded waking up each morning as bad news just got worse and worse. Given that my paper seemed to be at the ground zero of the event, I made the conscious decision to devote *New York Native* to covering every detail of the story. For the first two years our coverage was so thorough that some people started referring to my newspaper as "The New York Native Journal of Medicine." Many of our readers and advertisers resented our coverage and wanted us to focus on positive stories. But I felt that we had a responsibility get to the bottom of what was going on.

As the cases mounted and the gay community began to accept the reality of the epidemic, our coverage began to be appreciated and *New York Native* became a trusted source for the latest news about AIDS. In the April 25, 1985 issue of *Rolling Stone*, David Black said that *New York Native* deserved a Pulitzer Prize for our reporting. In his bestselling book, *And the Band Played On*, Randy Shilts wrote, "Because of the extraordinary reporting of the *New York Native*, the city's gay community had been exposed to far more information about AIDS than San Francisco in 1981 and 1982." And in the March 23, 1989 *Rolling Stone*, Katie Leishman wrote, "It is undeniable that many major AIDS stories were Ortleb's

6

months and sometimes years before mainstream journalists too them up." But that love affair with *New York Native* was about to end abruptly.

As I have detailed in my history of *New York Native*, *The Chronic Fatigue Syndrome Epidemic Cover-up*, as the epidemic went on and our reporting became more investigative, I began to notice serious credibility gaps in what the Centers for Disease Control was telling the public about the AIDS epidemic. AIDS increasingly reminded me of the period of egregious government mendacity that occurred during the Vietnam era. As the government began to build a paradigm around the notion that AIDS was caused by a retrovirus ultimately labelled "HIV," I watched as credible critics of the retroviral theory were silenced and vilified. I discuss the heroic voices that spoke out in *Peter Duesberg and the Duesbergians*.

My newspaper became even more controversial when we began reporting on another epidemic called Chronic Fatigue Syndrome. From our extensive reporting, it was hard not to conclude that Chronic Fatigue Syndrome is part of the AIDS epidemic and was linked to AIDS by a virus called HHV-6 which government scientists refused to take seriously.

As AIDS activists increasing lined up behind the government's HIV/AIDS paradigm and draconian public health agenda, the inconvenient truths my newspaper was reporting about HHV-6 and Chronic Fatigue Syndrome became increasingly unpopular. Nobody wanted to believe that the elite AIDS doctors and scientists might have gotten AIDS totally wrong. Act Up, New York's powerful AIDS activist group, voted to boycott *New York Native* and the did anything they could to put us out of business. Finally, in January 1997, we published our final issue.

In the last twenty years, I have given a great deal of thought to the nature of what happened to my newspaper and to the integrity of AIDS science and medicine. A number of my thoughts on the subject are collected in *Iatrogenocide: Notes for a Political Philosophy of Epidemiology and Science.* I have also written a play about the politics of the epidemic called *The Black Party.* My thoughts about the racial politics of AIDS can be found in a novella, *The Closing Argument.*

I have come to the conclusion that the similarities between AIDS science and Nazi science are too obvious for people of conscience to ignore. In his groundbreaking book about Nazi treatment of Jews, *"Life Unworthy of Life": Racial Phobia and Mass Murder in Hitler's Germany,* James M. Glass writes, "It was not cultural propagandists who organized the infamous 'special treatment' of the Jews; it was the public health officials, the scientific journals, the physicians, the administrators, and the lawyers, who feared the very presence of the Jews would endanger their families, their bodies, and ultimately their lives. To think of the Jew in such terms is insane from our perspective, but it was held to be sane in the culture caught up in the phobic projection of infection onto the Jews and the scientific authority legitimizing such beliefs." In many ways AIDS, or what I call "Holocaust II," involved what could be called "special epidemiological treatment" of the gays which was created and supported by health officials, scientific journals, physicians, administrators, lawyers, activists, celebrities, and many others. While the manner in which AIDS is understood by public health authorities and the general public is assumed to be sane, a closer look reveals that a genocidal insanity lurks beneath the surface. In the case of AIDS, a fraudulent and phobic epidemiology has been used to scapegoat and biomedically persecute the gay community. And many others.

In this chapter from The Chronic Fatigue Syndrome Epidemic Cover-up Volume Two, I discuss the scientist I consider to be among the important "architects" of Holocaust II. He played a key role in creating the kind of science which I describe in *Iatrogenocide* as being abnormal, totalitarian, and sociopathic.

I believe that when honest and brave scientists finally give Fauci's AIDS and Chronic Fatigue Syndrome work the due diligence it deserves, they will recognize that he has essentially been running a scientific Ponzi scheme for decades. Science now has its own Bernie Madoff.

Chronic Fatigue Syndrome and the HIV Ponzi Scheme

November 2, 1984 was an especially tragic day in the Chronic Fatigue Syndrome/AIDS epidemic. That was the day Anthony Fauci became the Director of the National Institutes of Allergy and Infectious Diseases. (NIAID). (*Good Intentions* p.128) It was the day a thin-skinned, physically ultra-diminutive man with a legendary Napoleonic attitude was positioned by destiny to become the de facto AIDS Czar. In the fog of culpability that constitutes what could be called "Holocaust II" one thing is clear: the buck, on its way to the very top of the government, at least pauses at the megalomaniac desk of Anthony Fauci.

In his book, *Good Intentions*, Bruce Nussbaum writes, "Fauci looked as if he had just stepped out of a limousine. Trim and athletic, Fauci's tailored suits, cuff-linked shirts, and aviator glasses set him far apart from the rest of the scientists and administrators at the NIH." (*GI* p.128) Fauci had risen quickly at NIH. According to Nussbaum, he began work at NIH in 1968 after his residency and "by 1977 he was deputy clinical director of NIAID." (*GI* p.128) Nussbaum describes Fauci as "an aggressive administrator," not a "details man," "a big picture kind of guy." (GI p.128) Nussbaum reports that "Fauci saw AIDS as a dreadful disease—and an opportunity for NIAID to grow into a much bigger, more powerful institute. AIDS was his big chance. He wasn't known as a brilliant scientist, and he had little background in managing a big bureaucracy; but Fauci did have ambition and drive to spare. This lackluster scientist was about to find his true vocation—empire building." (*GI* p.128) Unfortunately, the empire his extreme ambition

11

would build was "Holocaust II." If the mantra during Watergate was "follow the money," the mantra for uncovering the crimes of "Holocaust II" (other than "follow the heterosexism") could be "follow the empire building." And one of the morals of the story is that "lackluster" can have extreme consequences.

According to Nussbaum, in order to make his dreams come true, Fauci had to fight "for a bigger piece of the AIDS research pie" which he succeeded at by getting a sizable amount of the funds that Congress appropriated for AIDS research. (*GI* p.129) Fauci also had to fight to get AIDS out of the claws of the National Cancer Institute where the virus that was believed to be the cause of AIDS had been discovered (or, more accurately, stolen). Fauci argued that it was his institute's right to take on the lion's share of the research because, although AIDS did involve cancer (Kaposi's sarcoma), it was, after all, an infectious disease. Fauci got his way and his success is reflected in the evolving financial numbers Nussbaum provides: "A growing budget for AIDS research, like a rising tide, lifted Tony Fauci's profile considerably on the NIH campus. In 1982, NIAID received $297,000 in AIDS funding. In 1986 it received $63 million. In 1987, the sum reached $146 million. By 1990, NIAID's annual AIDS funding was pushing half a billion dollars. Tony Fauci's ship had come in." (*GI* p.132)

Fauci's ship coming in meant the gay community's would be sinking fast. It would fall to Anthony Fauci to be the Enforcer-in-Chief of the "homodemiological" HIV/AIDS and "Chronic Fatigue Syndrome is not AIDS" paradigms of "Holocaust II." No one can argue that he didn't do a spectacular job of paradigm enforcement for three dreadful decades.

Starting in the mid-1980s, an organization called the American Foundation for AIDS Research (amfAR) played a multifaceted role of raising money for HIV research and enlisting celebrities in a glamorous and ultimately shameful HIV propaganda campaign that made the putatively private organization essentially a de facto arm of the government's HIV/AIDS establishment. If one considers the HIV theory of AIDS a Potemkin biomedical village that gays were forced to live in, then amfAR as one of its leading real estate agents. John Lauritsen, in his book, *The AIDS War*, writes that "[amfAR] was founded as an alternative to the AIDS establishment, to provide funding for research that was *not* predicated on the 'AIDS virus' hypothesis. It didn't last long. . . . I am not aware that even a penny has ever been given to a researcher who publicly expressed doubts as to the etiological role of HIV or the benefits of the nucleoside analogues." (*AW* p.437)

In addition to becoming one of the leading private promoters of the government's HIV/AIDS paradigm propaganda, amfAR played a disturbing role in squelching serious scientific criticism of the HIV hypothesis and in helping turn the entire field of AIDS into a world of heterosexist, totalitarian, and abnormal science. Lauritsen describes an historically important amfAR moment in the AIDS disaster in his first book *Poison by Prescription*: "A 'Scientific Forum on the Etiology of AIDS,' sponsored by the American Foundation for AIDS Research (amfAR), was held on 9 April 1988 at the George Washington University in Washington, D.C. In the words of the amfAR 'fact sheet', the forum was convened to critically examine the evidence that human immunodeficiency virus (HIV) or other agents give rise to the disease complex known as AIDS." (*PBP* p.143)

According to Lauritsen, it was supposedly an opportunity for Peter Duesberg, the University of California at Berkeley retrovirologist who first challenged the HIV theory of AIDS "to confront members of the 'AIDS Establishment' over their hypothesis." (*PBP* p.143) He reports, however, that "Despite these praiseworthy intentions, the forum appears to have had a hidden agenda; to discredit Duesberg." (*PBP* p.143) Lauritsen characterized the forum as a "Kangaroo Court." The forum would make great scene in a play about the nasty, zany world of AIDS and HIV pseudoscience. It was anything but an honest, open collegial discussion about the nature of AIDS. Scientific philosopher Thomas Kuhn Kuhn would roll over in his grave if anyone called it genuinely scientific. By Kuhn's standards, some of the leading voices at the forum may have even demonstrated that they should not even have been considered real scientists. Politicians, yes, scientists not so much. Even the HIV theory's ardent acolyte, Michael Specter, the reporter from *The Washington Post* (and future *New Yorker* writer) who was among the 17 journalists at the Forum, saw through the charade, noting that the meeting "was billed as a scientific forum on the cause of AIDS but was really an attempt to put Duesberg's theories to rest." (*PBP* p.144) It was more like they wanted to put Duesberg himself permanently to rest.

The meeting had the tone and style that was endemic to HIV/AIDS research and characteristic of abnormal and totalitarian science. Lauritsen reported that "While no blows were struck, some of the HIV protagonists fell below the standards of civility that are expected in scholarly debate . . . . At all times Duesberg retained good manners and a sense of humor, in the face of invective, insults, and clowning from his opponents." (*PBP* p.144)

One of the signs that AIDS in general was being conducted in the opposite world of what could be called abnormal, totalitarian science was the uncanny willingness of the scientists to abandon the traditional rules of evidence known as Koch's postulates. Instead, AIDS researchers, including the ones at the amfAR forum, were willing to "revise Koch's in a more permissive direction: it would no longer be necessary to find the microbe in all cases of the disease. Mere correlations between microbial *antibodies* and the progression of the disease would be sufficient. HIV could be proved 'epidemiologically' to be the cause of AIDS." (*PBP* p.145) Given the unrecognized sexual politics of the science that was operative among this crowd, they were basically saying, without realizing it, that causation could be established *"homodemiologically."* The presumptions of heterosexist and political epidemiology would trump the traditional rules of evidence. And those rules could basically be summed up as "Heads I win and tails you lose." "You" basically being gays and eventually blacks.

Lauritsen caught the powerful HIV advocates in the act of doublespeak that is common to abnormal, totalitarian science: "Actually, the HIV advocates talked out of both sides of their mouths with regard to Koch's postulates. On the one hand, they disparaged them as in need of 'modification' (read abandonment); on the other hand, they were doing their best to come up with data that would satisfy at least the first postulate." (*PBP* p.145)

Duesberg's opponents at the forum included a living, breathing example of scientific conflict of interest, William Haseltine, a scientist who was in the process of making a lot of money from HIV testing, and Anthony Fauci, the empire-building Director of NIAID.

At the amfAR Forum, Fauci and others played a curious unfair game with Duesberg. Hypocritically they accused Duesberg of citing research that was out of date even though it was basically *the same research quoted at that time* by the AIDS establishment. On the other hand, when Duesberg would ask Fauci and others for actual references to support *their* statements at the amfAR forum, he was "rudely rebuffed," and according to Lauritsen, they tried to shore up their viewpoint about HIV with unpublished data, or "their own private facts." (*PBP* p.147) "Private facts" not on the public record are another sure sign that AIDS was a manifestation of the opposite world of abnormal, totalitarian and sociopathic science. Unfortunately, their private facts about AIDS were also connected to each other by a private scientific logic.

The 800-pound gorilla at the amfAR forum was the fact that evidence of HIV could *not be found in all AIDS patients*, which should have been strong—damning even—evidence that HIV couldn't possibly be the cause of AIDS, that is, if Kuhnian normal science was being practiced. As scientist Marcel Beluda pointed out at the meeting, "sometimes even a single exception is sufficient to disprove a theory." . . . This is the crux of the matter. The virus cannot be found in all cases of AIDS." (*PBP* p.151) One could say that still believing that HIV is the cause of AIDS in the face of evidence that it could not be found in all patients is Exhibit A that delusion and denial were running the show.

Fauci's answer belongs in a beginner's textbook on the card tricks of abnormal science: "Fauci responded to Beluda by saying that a good lab was able to isolate the virus in 90-100% of the cases, that there was 'no question about it.' Fauci did not provide a reference to published data, nor did he indicate what the 'good labs' were, or how exactly they differed from the not-so-good labs." (*PBP* p.151) References belong to the abandoned Kuhnian world of normal science.

Duesberg made a number of arguments, based on his years as one of the celebrated deans of retroviral research, about why HIV could not possibly be the cause of AIDS.

Lauritsen wrote that Fauci's presentation "while aspiring to be a point-by-point rebuttal to Duesberg, consisted mainly of disconnected assertions, delivered in a tone of petulant indignation. Epidemiological studies conducted in San Francisco and unpublished laboratory reports seemed to be the basis of most of his statements. So far as I could tell, he understood none of Duesberg's arguments . . . ." (*PBP* p.155)

The role of the AIDS politics of epidemiology in AIDS research showed itself dramatically at the forum. According to Lauritsen, "In the question period, Beluda asked if the evidence were sufficient that HIV is necessary for the development of AIDS, Fauci replied that he hoped the epidemiologists would answer that question." (*PBP* p.157) (Given the political and heterosexist nature of AIDS epidemiology, one could guess how *that* was going to turn out.)

The most shocking and downright hilarious episode at the forum occurred when Harvard Medical School's William Haseltine spoke. Lauritsen reported that "His presentation was devoted largely to personal attacks on Duesberg." (*PBP* p.157) Ironically, *he* accused Duesberg of resorting to personal attacks. In another telltale moment of abnormal and totalitarian science, Lauritsen caught Haseltine trying to explain away the anomalies about the evidence of AIDS in men and women in America: "He attacked Duesberg's 'paradox,' that the AIDS virus seemed to be able to discriminate between boys and girls, by saying that this was not true outside the U.S.—in Africa, about equal numbers of men and women develop AIDS. (He seemed oblivious to the paradox that a microbe should be able to discriminate in one country, but not in another.)" (*PBP* p.158) In a memorable moment that perfectly captured the essence of the past and future of AIDS research, Haseltine showed the audience a slide of a graph that was meant to absolutely demolish Duesberg's argument. The slide was supposed to show a correlation between the rise in HIV titers with the decline of T cells in the progression of AIDS. There was just one small problem: Duesberg quickly noticed that *there were no units on the vertical axis of the slide.* Haseltine was angry and flustered by the charge and had to ask **Dr. Robert Redfield**, an AIDS researcher from the military, how the slide was prepared. At the forum Redfield said, "different measurements were used," but later that night at a post-forum party, according to Lauritsen's report, Redfield told Duesberg and other people at the gathering that "the graph had been prepared to illustrate a theoretical possibility. It had no units on it for the simple reason that *it was not based on any data at all.* In other words, the slide was a fake." (*PBP* p.161) That's the kind of ideology-based data that was used to back up the HIV theory of AIDS which changed the course of millions of lives and fostered the HHV-6 catastrophe.

In terms of the habitual use of political epidemiology (or "homodemiology") rather than real science to deal with AIDS during "Holocaust II," the most disturbing talk was given by **Warren Winkelstein**, Professor of Biomedical Environmental Health Sciences at U.C. Berkeley. Essentially, he too suggested that AIDS would require *a new kind of science.* According to Lauritsen, "the point of Winkelstein's presentation is that Koch's postulates should be superseded by new standards for establishing the causal relationship between microbes and disease, and that these standards should be based upon 'epidemiology' or, as it were, correlations of various kinds." (*PBP* p.162) If this crowd had superseded traditional science any more than they did, we all would probably be dead. (But wait. There is still time.)

Most of the scientific world was not aware of the degree to which this zany cast of characters was improvising a questionable newfangled science as they went along. And it was being done in a Fauci-style of "petulant indignation," to reprise Lauritsen's very apt phrase. That it was all dependent on a loosey-goosey, all too subjective political "discipline" like epidemiology should have disturbed Lauritsen's sixteen journalistic colleagues who were at the amfAR affair. But there was already a tragically cozy relationship between the media and the abnormal, totalitarian and sociopathic scientists of "Holocaust II." For three decades as the HIV/AIDS paradigm held sway, most of the reporters who covered AIDS were a self-satisfied, inattentive, group-thinking, intellectually slothful bunch who wouldn't know independent, journalistic due diligence if it bit them. A corrupt scientific community could totally depend on them.

Lauritsen's eyewitness record of the forum (originally published in *New York Native*) was an important contribution to the history of the flakey beginnings of the science and totalitarian politics of AIDS. His diligent and critical reporting is proof that *not every journalist* was hoodwinked by these charlatans. He didn't buy into this new improvised epidemiological science that the AIDS establishment was dumping on the public: "I do not accept the proposition that Koch's postulates should be abandoned in favor of epidemiological correlations. This would be a step backward, a step away from scientific rigor, a step towards impressionism and confusion." (*PBP* p.162) Lauritsen didn't acknowledge it, but it was also a big heterosexist (and ultimately racist) step backwards.

Like many others, Lauritsen came face to face with totalitarian, abnormal, and sociopathic science. Unfortunately, even though he was openly gay himself, he didn't grasp the manner in which the infernal game was being played—or what the game was actually concealing. He didn't fully perceive the homodemiological underpinnings of what was happening before his very eyes. But he definitely grasped the fact that the science of the budding AIDS Establishment was utterly bogus. He concluded his report by writing "I am more convinced than ever that HIV is not the cause of AIDS. If the HIV advocates were sure of their hypothesis, they would want to enlighten Duesberg and the rest of us; they would want to publish their arguments in a proper scientific journal complete with references. They would not need to resort to stonewalling, deception, and personal abuse." (*PBP* p.168) Science had been supplanted by totalitarian petulance.

The 1988 amfAR Forum was another one of the tragic "What if?" moments in the dark history of AIDS. What if the reporters had looked closer at Haseltine's fake slide and realized that it was the tip of the iceberg, a little like the scientific version of the Watergate break-in that would have led them to a much bigger crime if they only followed the lies? What if they had reported that AIDS science, as practiced by Anthony Fauci, was simply out-to-lunch? What if they had been independent enough to notice that epidemiology was overplaying its arrogant, biased hand and that, in reality, it is actually a soft, subjective enterprise vulnerable to political manipulation? Why was it beyond the pale to wonder if this defensive and cranky gathering was actually the expression of some rather unsavory feelings and hostilities directed at the so-called beneficiaries of this new kind of "science," namely the gay community? Maybe someone should have asked if there was something funky about a group of hostile, arrogant, white heterosexual mostly-male scientists performing their jerry-built kind of seat-of-the-pants epidemiological science on gays. Wasn't that a formula for all kinds of prurient, heterosexist pseudoscientific mischief if ever there was one? In terms of majorities doing their science on minorities, hadn't anyone ever heard of Nazi science or the Tuskegee Syphilis Experiment? God only knows what personal sexual issues were being acted out by this elite motley crew under the cover of what has turned out to be highfalutin retroviral

20

claptrap. Why didn't anyone other than Lauritsen notice the peculiar, unscientific defensiveness of the whole affair, i.e. that the ladies had protested too much? And most importantly for the main event, why was HHV-6, which had been discovered in AIDS patients two years before that curious amfAR forum, not put on the table for discussion?

Fauci believed in the kind of transparency and communications with the public that are typical of abnormal science. He laid out the draconian media policy that he would maintain for the nearly thirty years he ran the totalitarian HIV/AIDS empire in a brief piece he wrote for the AAAS Observer on September 1, 1989.

Fauci wrote, "When I first got involved in AIDS research, I was reluctant to deal with the press. I thought it was not dignified. But there was a lot of distortion by those who were speaking to the press so I changed my mind." The "distortion" was, of course, coming from those who didn't agree with the very dignified Fauci about the etiology of AIDS. Fauci had his own idea of what the media's responsibility is. He notes that his interpretation of what the media is supposed to do "doesn't even jibe with what competent journalists think." He asserts that the big dilemma for journalists is between what is "important" and what is "newsworthy" and he notes that they sometimes "are not the same." He whines about the fact that journalists are more interested in the latest story of a cure than the "magnificent science" involving the regulatory genes of HIV.

Fauci describes what he thinks is the hierarchy of media. It ranges from *The New York Times* and *The Washington Post* all the way down to publications that "care only about sales or have axes to grind." (He had yet to face the unwashed barbarians of the blogs and the commenters of the online forums.) One can safely assume that the publications with axes to grind were the ones who didn't agree with the axe that the petulant Fauci himself was grinding.

It is amusing that Fauci pontificated in 1989 that "the media are no place for amateurs, particularly when talking about a public health problem of the magnitude of AIDS." Especially when one considers the magnitude of the HHV-6 public health problem that this very self-reverential scientist (that Bruce Nussbaum described as "lackluster") himself helped create for the whole human race. While Fauci would make one think that the real problem in AIDS journalism was the clownish journalist who can't spell "retrovirus" or one who didn't listen carefully after asking questions, his real quarry in this peevish little piece is something far more serious. Fauci's real problem was journalists who not only *could* spell "retrovirus" but could also actually hear what he was saying *all too well*. The kind of journalists who also knew things about retroviruses and listened to what he was saying so closely and critically that they could make life unpleasant for Fauci and his powerful AIDS cronies by asking inconvenient questions.

Fauci's nose should have grown several feet when he wrote, "We know that reporters must consult more than a single source and make room for dissenting opinions." What was yet to come in the AAAS piece made that one of the biggest fibs in the history of American science. Under the pretense of giving us a little lesson in the relationship between science and the media and warning that people too often believe what they read in the papers, Fauci reveals his real agenda: "One striking example is Peter Duesberg's theory that HIV is not the cause of AIDS. I laughed at that for a while, but it led to a lot of public concern that HIV was a hoax. The theory had a great deal of credibility just on the basis of news coverage." This was Fauci being intellectually dishonest on a couple of counts. Duesberg never said it was a *hoax*. He said it was a *mistake*. A hoax is a whole other ball of wax, and it is an example of using language politically to deliberately misrepresent the opposition. Duesberg wasn't saying something similar to those who say that the landing on the moon was just staged with props and a camera. He was a Nobel-caliber expert on retroviruses pointing out the deficiencies of the HIV theory in AIDS using basic logic and analyzing the available evidence. And blaming the media for the credibility given to Duesberg's ideas ignored all the scientists, (eventually including two Nobel Prize winners), who publicly supported Duesberg's skepticism. Fauci was Trumpian in that he was essentially accusing those who spotted his fake science as being purveyors of fake news.

Fauci then introduces us to the smarter member of his family, his sister: "My barometer of what the general public is thinking is my sister Denise. My sister Denise is an intelligent woman who reads avidly, listens to the radio, and watches television, but she is not a scientist. When she calls me and questions my integrity as a scientist, there really is a problem. Denise has called me at least ten times about Peter Duesberg. She says, 'Anthony'—she is the only one who calls me Anthony, 'are you sure he's wrong?' That's the power of putting someone on television or in the press, although there is virtually nothing in his argument that makes any scientific sense." This captures how touchy Fauci was. No one was questioning his "integrity as a scientist." His sister was simply asking him if it was *possible* that he was wrong, and the answer that would have shown some scientific integrity would have been, "Yes, my dear Denise, it is always possible that I'm wrong, although I think the evidence suggests I'm right." The fact that Fauci took this *soooooo* personally speaks volumes about the petulant chip-on-the-shoulder attitude problems of those in charge of AIDS. Fauci put it all on the line. Questioning his so-called science was a threat to his very being. It shouldn't surprise anyone that he was willing to

23

viciously fight for so long during "Holocaust II" to keep everyone from seeing what a house of cards he had helped build. The funny thing is that in a number of ways this scientific masterpiece suggests he *did* have serious problems in the integrity department. (Between the lines of the piece Freudian historians may one day even find the glimmer of a guilty conscience.)

Fauci, like most of the crowd that gave us "Holocaust II," knew only too well what normal, nontotalitarian science is supposed to look like: "People are especially confused when they see divergent viewpoints about the same thing. They do not understand that the beauty of science is that it is self-corroborating and self-correcting, that it is important for scientists to be wrong." (If that's really the case, Fauci *was* indeed doing something incredibly important with HIV.) It was actually Fauci who didn't understand that the whole process of self-corroboration and self-correction was being short-circuited by the totalitarian hijinks of the touchy HIV/AIDS establishment that was growing more dominant by the day. The very tone of Fauci's piece, its extraordinary imperiousness and presumptuousness about the stupidity of the public, points to the fundamental problem for a society in which arrogant and dishonest elite scientific communities have more and more power. Fauci would not only be the judge and jury of what was true in science, but he also wanted to decide *who* deserved to write about it and *what* they should write. He clearly left no room for the possibility that the really good journalists would be the kind that questioned what *he* had to say.

Fauci also made it pretty clear in the piece that, try as they might, AIDS critics and dissidents would get absolutely nowhere because he was permanently stacking the deck against them: "The lack of clear-cut black-or-white answers plagues the biomedical sciences compared with the physical sciences. Stanley Pons and Martin Fleishmann said they had achieved nuclear fusion at room temperature. Other scientists tried, but they could not reproduce it. Bingo it's over. But because we cannot ethically do clinical trials to establish that he is wrong, I am probably going to be answering Peter Duesberg for the rest of my life." Someone near him should have tried to convince Fauci that it wasn't all about *him*. One also loves the presumption that he was going to control the official etiology of AIDS *for the rest of his life*. Unfortunately, *he almost has*. Beyond the breathtaking megalomania of the statement is the stupidity that the only way to show HIV wasn't the cause of AIDS was to do clinical trials with patients. All it would have taken would have been a few patients with AIDS *who had no evidence of HIV*. The only people that would be hurt by the implications of that finding would be the dishonest and incompetent scientists, like Fauci, whose undeserved reputations and incomes had depended upon the HIV theory. Those HIV-negative patients would be forthcoming—in spades. In fact those patients were basically the very immune-compromised Chronic Fatigue Syndrome patients a doctor named Richard DuBois had seen in his Atlanta practice *before* the socio-epidemiological construction of the heterosexist and racist HIV/AIDS paradigm.

Hillary Johnson reported on the DuBois Atlanta cases in *Osler's Web: Inside the Labyrinth of Chronic Fatigue Syndrome Epidemic*, her epic work of journalism detailing the CDC's failure to acknowledge the true nature of the Chronic Fatigue Syndrome epidemic. It is now all too painfully obvious that the DuBois cases—with the telltale signs of hypergammaglobulinemia, t-cell perturbations and persistent reactivated EBV and CMV infections—were the beginning of the real AIDS/CFS/HHV-6 disaster. According to Johnson, in 1980 Richard DuBois "saw a thirteen-year old girl who suffered from a seemingly endless case of mono. As the months passed, he identified several more cases of the curious syndrome in his practice." (OW p.7) He wasn't alone. Johnson reported that he was in touch with other clinicians who had seen similar cases and he and his colleagues eventually had a research article published about it in the Southern Medical Journal in 1984, the same year the big consequential government mistake of certifying HIV as the official AIDS virus occurred. According to Johnson, "they [DuBois and his colleagues] had believed that they were describing a new syndrome, one that would have increasing importance and was worthy of national attention." (OW p.7) The DuBois patients morphed into the millions of Chronic Fatigue Syndrome and HHV-6 patients that Fauci and his organization (which was supposed to handle infectious diseases) were willfully ignoring while building their Potemkin HIV/AIDS empire.

At the end of Fauci's little *AAAS* piece comes the shot across the media's bow from the tiny AIDS czar: "Scientists need to get more sophisticated about expressing themselves. But the media have to do their homework. They have got to learn the issues and the background. And they should realize that their accuracy is noted by the scientific community. Journalists who make too many mistakes, who are sloppy, are going to find that their access to scientists may diminish." In other words, the scientists that journalists reported on were going to be the high-handed and underhanded final arbiters of what the public knows about science. They could decide to cut off journalists *they* defined as making mistakes and being sloppy, and one would assume that one of those sloppy mistakes would probably entail giving any coverage to scientists like Peter Duesberg, who raised serious questions about what was being called good science by Fauci and the rest of the HIV/AIDS establishment. Fauci was basically

26

saying that he and his cronies would only be accountable to themselves which is the hermetically-sealed, closed-community essence of should be called totalitarian, abnormal, and ultimately sociopathic science.

If anyone ever makes a serious film about "Holocaust II" it will have to include the shocking revelation (already referred to above) that came to light during the Eighth International Conference on AIDS in Amsterdam during July of 1992. Its historic importance rivals that of the Wannsee conference during World War II or the Gulf of Tonkin incident. It was *the moment of no turning back*, the moment a fateful line was crossed, a life of virtual pseudoscientific crime against humanity was virtually signed onto and those responsible for "Holocaust II" lost all forms of plausible deniability. AIDS almost overnight became AIDSgate and a very unique Nazi-like biomedical and epidemiological assault against humanity. And, ultimately, the man who stood at the center of the developments that came out of Amsterdam was Anthony Fauci. Before Amsterdam one might be able to say that Fauci wasn't exactly the Bernie Madoff of the biomedical Ponzi Scheme that maintained AIDS, Chronic Fatigue Syndrome and the HHV-6 spectrum catastrophe. *But not after Amsterdam.*

Hillary Johnson provided a detailed account of what happened at that Amsterdam conference in her book. She recounts how the conference was electrified by news from a small press conference that was held in California at which a scientist named "Subhir Gupta, a University of California immunologist, reported he had isolated particles of a previously unknown retrovirus from an HIV-negative, ailing sixty-six-year-old woman, her symptomless daughter and six other patients." (*OW* p.600) According to Johnson, "Investigators and the lay press gathered in Holland were riveted by Gupta's announcement that the older woman suffered from an 'AIDS-like' condition wherein a component of her immune system, a subset of T-cells called CD4 cells, were severely depleted. In addition, she had suffered a bout of *Pneumocystis carinii* pneumonia, a so-called opportunistic infection that afflicted many AIDS patients whose CD4 cells were depleted." (*OW* p.600)

That announcement was soon outdone by a flurry of shocking revelations from additional scientists at the Amsterdam conference who had "findings of retrovirus particles in HIV-negative patients with AIDS-like symptoms." (*OW* p.601) A near panic was almost set off internationally by the possibility that there was a second previously unrecognized AIDS epidemic on the horizon that was caused by a non-HIV agent. (*OW* p.601)

According to Johnson, it turned out that the Centers for Disease Control *was already aware* of such HIV-negative cases of an AIDS-like illness. (*OW* p.601) Johnson reported that months before Gupta's press conference two CDC scientists had reported on "six cases of non-HIV positive AIDS." (*OW* p.601) Their conclusion was that "HIV may not be the only infectious cause of immune deficiency." (*OW* p.601) Two AIDS viruses? A gay one and a straight one? OMG!

The HIV-negative cases of AIDS-like illness set off an explosion in the press, most notably from Lawrence Altman, the reporter who guided *The New York Times* dreadful, sycophantic reporting on AIDS throughout "Holocaust II." In the *Times* Altman wrote that the CDC's embarrassment was "huge because the agency had lost control over the dissemination of new information in the field of AIDS." (*OW* p.602) (That anyone at the *Times* could stress the importance of a government agency *controlling information* with a straight face is pretty amazing and revealing.)

According to Johnson, the CFS research community was especially fascinated by the fact that the Gupta HIV-negative

AIDS-like cases were Chronic Fatigue Syndrome sufferers. (*OW* p.604) And for anyone following the bizarre scientific politics of AIDS, it was interesting that Gupta's colleague, the man who supposedly isolated the new retrovirus was none other than Zaki Salahuddin, the scientist who had worked for Robert Gallo and had faced criminal charges for creating a company that garnered illegal self-dealt income from his position at the National Cancer Institute. Johnson reported that when Salahuddin was asked whether HIV-negative AIDS might be Chronic Fatigue Syndrome, he said, "It's a fair statement. But I'm not a prophet. Time and money [are] required for this." (*OW* p.604) Johnson also reported, "Salahuddin confirmed that he and Gupta, who had a cohort of CFS patients in his clinical practice and who had presented papers on the immunology of CFS at medical conferences on the disease, had discussed the possibility that CFS and non-HIV positive AIDS were the same disease." (*OW* p.604) Also, according to Johnson, the non-HIV positive AIDS cases caught the attention of Paul Cheney, one of the two pioneering Lake Tahoe Chronic Fatigue Syndrome researchers. Johnson wrote, "For years he had observed that some CFS patients met the government's defining criteria for AIDS on every count except infection with human immunodeficiency virus." (*OW* p.604) He also told Johnson that "It was hardly unheard of . . . to diagnose the kinds of opportunistic infections that torment AIDS victims—maladies like thrush, candida and pneumonia—in CFS." (*OW* p.604) In the world of normal science this would have been called "the smoking gun."

The AIDS conference in 1992 should have been one of those great moments in normal science as described by Thomas Kuhn. It could have been a moment when disturbing "anomalies" should have attracted the "attention of a scientific community." (*The Structure of Scientific Revolutions* p.ix) But this would not be a moment for AIDS research that "the profession can no longer evade anomalies that subvert the existing tradition of scientific practice" which would "begin the extraordinary investigations that lead the profession at last to a new set of commitments, a new basis for the practice of science." (*SSR* p.6) This would *not* be one of those eureka moments in science characterized by "the community's rejection of one time-honored scientific theory in favor of another incompatible with it." (*SSR* p.6) There would be no "transformation of the world within which science was done." (*SSR* p.6) There would be no "change in the rules governing the prior practice." (*SSR* p.7) As a result of what happened in Amsterdam, scientists would *not* alter their "conception of entities with which [they] had long been familiar." (*SSR* p.7) Amsterdam would *not* cause the AIDS researchers' worlds to be "qualitatively transformed as well as quantitatively enriched by fundamental novelties of either fact or theory." (*SSR* p.7) After the revelations of HIV-negative AIDS cases, the researchers would still *not* give up their "shared paradigm." (*SSR* p.11) No new AIDS (or Chronic Fatigue Syndrome = AIDS) paradigm was allowed to reveal itself in Amsterdam and subsequently be fairly examined and debated. The HIV-negative cases of AIDS would *not* be recognized as an important scientific surprise that would lead scientists "to see nature in a different way." (*SSR* p.53) The scientific world of AIDS researchers did not change "in an instant" (*SSR* p.56) the way it might have if AIDS research was taking place in the world of normal science. (And consequently, immune-system-destroying HHV-6 would remain locked in the basement of "science.")

Tragically, the HIV-negative AIDS cases were not a wake-up call for the scientists that "something had gone wrong" and hence the anomalous cases were not "a prelude to discovery." (*SSR* p.57) Even though the HIV-negative

AIDS cases "violated deeply entrenched expectations," (*SSR* p.59) they were not allowed to change *anything* about the AIDS paradigm. In Kuhn's world of normal science, the "traditional pursuit prepares the way for its own change.' (*SSR* p.65) Amsterdam showed that AIDS research was being conducted in normal science's cockamamie opposite world, one that should be called "abnormal, totalitarian and sociopathic science." Even if the HIV-negative AIDS cases could have ultimately led to a new paradigm that was "able to account for wider range of natural phenomena," (*SSR* p.66) they were dead on arrival. No "novel theory" about AIDS which was a "direct response to crisis" (*SSR* p.75) was allowed to emerge because the abnormal, totalitarian, and sociopathic science of AIDS was *politically invulnerable* to crisis. At that historic conference there was never any chance that the HIV/AIDS theory would be "declared invalid" even though a new "CFS is a form of AIDS" paradigm was staring out at the conference from the new anomalous data and was a perfectly credible "alternate candidate." (*SSR* p.77) Kuhn wrote that the decision to reject one paradigm is always simultaneously the decision to accept another, and the judgment leading to that decision involves the comparison of both paradigms with nature and with each other." (*SSR* p.77) The HIV-negative AIDS cases were *not allowed* to catalyze that kind of fertile intellectual process in Amsterdam. Kuhn would probably argue that absent a new paradigm to examine and accept in Amsterdam, there was no exit from the HIV/AIDS paradigm because "To reject one paradigm without simultaneously substituting another is to reject science itself." (*SSR* p.79) In a way, much of what happened at the AIDS conference was based on appeals to something quite characteristic of the AIDS establishment and abnormal science: *authority*. The petulant HIV/AIDS authorities basically said, "Nothing here, folks. Please move along." And unfortunately, the scientific community and the media (with a few notable exceptions) did exactly that. Kuhnian *anomaly* didn't turn into Kuhnian *crisis* and that in turn did not explode into Kuhnian *scientific revolution* as it should have. The HIV-negative cases in Amsterdam should have led to a period of what Kuhn called "extraordinary science" (*SSR* p.82) in which "the rules of normal science become increasingly blurred." (*SSR* p.83) (Although one could argue that the rules of AIDS research already actually were a shocking chocolate mess.) Amsterdam would not be the transformative moment when "formerly standard solutions of solved problems are called into question." (*SSR* p.83) The conference should have been a fruitful time when scientists were "terribly confused." (*SSR* p.84) If things had gone the way they should have at that conference, the assembled AIDS researchers would have ultimately changed their view of "the field, its methods, and its goals." (*SSR* p.85) HHV-6 might have been allowed to reveal itself in all its pathological glory. And the scientists who had given us the HIV paradigm would have been revealed in all their vainglory.

Had the science of Amsterdam been *normal*, both AIDS research and Chronic Fatigue Syndrome research might have morphed into one unified discipline. The dismantling of the "Chronic Fatigue Syndrome isn't AIDS" paradigm should have begun in earnest. HHV-6 (and its spectrum or family) might have emerged quickly as the unifying viral agent(s) of those two epidemics which should have always been considered one in the first place. And those two epidemics were just the tip of the HHV-6 iceberg. What happened in Amsterdam was a virtual nosological and epidemiological crime. It was the deliberate attempt to use *sheer political force* to make a legitimate scientific crisis disappear. As a result, scientists would not turn to what Kuhn describes as a "philosophical analysis as a device for unlocking the riddles

32

of their field." (*SSR* p.88) "Philosophical analysis" was Greek to this confederacy of dunces. The crisis was not allowed to play itself out and would not loosen what Kuhn calls the "stereotypes" and provide "the incremental data necessary for a fundamental paradigm shift." (*SSR* p.89) There would be no Kuhnian "transition from normal to extraordinary research." (*SSR* p.91) It should have been painfully clear in Amsterdam "that an existing paradigm [had] ceased to function adequately in the exploration of an aspect of nature to which that paradigm itself had previously led the way." (*SSR* p.92)

A potentially life-saving scientific revolution in AIDS and CFS research was politically nipped in the bud in Amsterdam and in the months that followed. No "new theory" was allowed to surface that would "permit predictions that are different from those derived from its predecessor" (*SSR* p.97) Kuhn asserted that "the price of significant scientific advance is a commitment that runs the risk of being wrong."(*SSR* p.101) Those in control of the abnormal science of AIDS had no interest in engaging in *any* kind of science that would prove *them* wrong. "Wrong" was not in their cultish vocabulary. They had bet their white heterosexual male professional reputations and the credibility of American science on their ridiculous and dangerous HIV/AIDS and "Chronic Fatigue Syndrome is not AIDS" paradigms. Fake dividends of their scientific Ponzi Scheme would be paid out for decades.

What happened in Amsterdam was the opening and almost simultaneously closing of a Pandora's Box of incredibly important scientific questions and implications. The person most responsible for keeping that box closed then and for the next two decades was the de facto AIDS Czar, the tantrum-prone Anthony Fauci. This may have been the last chance for Fauci and the HIV/AIDS establishment to turn back from the precipice of the HHV-6 spectrum catastrophe. But even his sister Denise could not save him from securing this dark place in history.

According to Hillary Johnson, "On August 15, federal scientists convened a meeting in Atlanta to discuss the emerging health threat of non-HIV positive AIDS. In the three weeks since Sudhir Gupta's paper on his isolation of a new intracisternal retrovirus in a handful of cases, the number of reported cases had risen from approximately thirty to fifty. Nobel prize winners, members of the National Academy of Sciences, CDC's AIDS administrators, and Anthony Fauci, head of the National Institute of Allergy and Infectious Diseases, formed a panel to query scientists Gupta, David Ho of the Aaron Diamond AIDS Center in New York and Jeffrey Laurence, a Cornell Medical College cancer and AIDS specialist and associate professor of medicine, each of whom had been studying cases of the syndrome and discovered evidence of retroviral infection in patients." (*OW* p.606) It didn't matter how many brilliant scientists from different institutions were queried at the meeting, because their mindsets about HIV were all the same. It was like a mini-Woodstock of groupthink. There was no turning back from the HIV/AIDS and "Chronic Fatigue Syndrome *is not* AIDS" paradigm. The carved-in-stone paradigm was eight years old at that point and the nation's heterosexist and racist AIDS propaganda and public health policies had been built on its assumptions. The gay and black communities had been herded into it like cattle into a train. It was another moment in abnormal science in which the privileged and paranoid foxes had formed a panel to investigate the henhouse.

The manner in which Fauci and his colleagues basically covered up the shocking anomalies of HIV-negative AIDS was relatively simple and Orwellian: as previously noted, they disingenuously gave the HIV-negative cases an obfuscatory new name (Idiopathic CD4 T lymphocytopenia or ICL) and they insisted by fiat that they were not really AIDS cases. The HIV/AIDS elite insisted that because there was no unifying geographic or chronological "risk factor" (OW P.603) to be found in these ordinary Americans and they shared no official AIDS risk factors, there was no HIV-negative AIDS or AIDS-like epidemic covertly occurring in the general population. Fauci's concerned sister Denise would not have to lose sleep at night.

Because the "Chronic Fatigue Syndrome *is not* AIDS" paradigm was not challenged by what happened at the Amsterdam Conference in 1992, for at least another two more decades, the Chronic Fatigue Syndrome patients were locked into their pathetic heterosexist wild goose chase to find a cause while constantly avoiding the obvious links between their medical issues and AIDS. They had Tony Fauci's blessing for that fool's errand. His basic attitude toward CFS was that people shouldn't be ashamed of being told that their problem was psychiatric, (*OW* p.334) which was how the disease was deceptively framed by the government for nearly three decades. And of course, they were just the canaries in the HHV-6 mine. Everyone suffering from multi-systemic problems of the HHV-6 spectrum (like multiple sclerosis, fibromyalgia, autism, and even Morgellons) would ultimately pay a heavy price for the intellectual dishonesty and legerdemain of the 1992 AIDS conference.

Fauci and his colleagues told the public that the HIV-negative cases of AIDS-like illness were rare, but of course it all depended on disease definitions and *who* was doing the defining and counting. Fauci disingenuously sent out a call that summer asking that all HIV-negative cases be reported immediately *to him*. An editorial in *New York Native* heeded his call: "Last week Anthony Fauci of the National Institute of Allergy and Infectious Diseases asked that all cases of HIV-negative AIDS be reported to him. We reported thirteen million American cases. That's the estimate of the number of cases of Chronic Fatigue and Immune Dysfunction, a condition that research (if anyone bothers to read it) suggests is essentially HIV-negative AIDS." (*OW* p.605)

The editorial had no impact on Anthony Fauci and it would not be the only time he would ignore the *New York Native* during "Holocaust II."

One could ultimately say that Denise Fauci's petulant brother himself represented one of the most significant scientific paradigm shifts, one that moved the whole world from normal to abnormal, totalitarian, and sociopathic science. During the Fauci years, The Age of Scientific Racketeering began in earnest. Bernie Madoff has a twin in science whose Ponzi Scheme is a gift that keeps on giving.

Afterword

Scientific totalitarianism is the background music of Anthony Fauci's brilliant and long-lasting Ponzi scheme. A so-called liberal democracy like America demands a covert form of scientific totalitarianism that does not scare the horses of oversight and public opinion. Fauci knew how to manipulate the levers of institutional power and image-making in ways that Bernie Madoff would envy. For a scientific Ponzi scheme to prevail in America and Europe, nobody must recognize that they have acquiesced to a major medical and scientific fraud. Doctors must follow protocols established by the HIV/AIDS Ponzi scheme and patients must not question them. Sanctions should stand at the ready if they do. Nobody must see the telltale signs of fraud, deceit, and censorship. Fauci knew the tricks required to turn ivy-league-educated elite journalists into servile puppets and perky stenographers. I coined the term "Bob Club" to describe the sycophantic journalists who enabled the massive scientific fraud of disgraced National Cancer Institute researcher Robert Gallo. The "Tony Club" is even worse and consequential in ways that will take medical historians generations to fully illuminate. A long list of servile journalists who were chummy with Fauci and enabled his Ponzi scheme will have a lot to answer for. An intimidating voice, a good haircut, and suits that fit well go a long way in science especially if you are as skilled in the art of veiled and not-so-veiled threats as Fauci is.

Laziness is not a Fauci flaw. It took a great deal of industriousness to cover up the role of the HHV-6/7/8 family viruses in "AIDS," Chronic Fatigue Syndrome and a myriad of immune disorders that constitute the real "AIDS" epidemic that the Ponzi scheme conceals from the public. To keep the entire NIH establishment from dealing with Chronic Fatigue Syndrome and its relationship to AIDS for almost four decades took a great deal of persistent effort.

Fauci is not stupid. There is no way that some part of him didn't recognize that serious Chronic Fatigue Syndrome research would have easily brought down his whole HIV house of cards if it had been officially acknowledged. Even noting publicly that it was uncanny the way any little bit of Chronic Fatigue Syndrome research (and there is tons of it) showed the illness was similar to AIDS would have threatened the Fauci Ponzi scheme. The HIV house of cards and the wall that separates AIDS and Chronic Fatigue Syndrome are the Fauci legacy. The recognition that he got AIDS wrong because he got Chronic Fatigue Syndrome wrong and vice versa would have turned him into an instant disgrace in the eyes of his family and friends. The egregious self-esteem he had carefully nurtured from his early days in Brooklyn would be a plate of Bethesda toast.

In my career as the publisher of *New York Native* (1980-1997), I had one phone conversation with Anthony Fauci in which I heard his petulance and thin-skinned nature in real time. I called him after I had written an editorial that was critical of Fauci in the form of a satirical poem. As readers probably already suspect, Dr. Fauci does not have much of a sense of humor. Especially when it is directed at him by someone in the media who does not know their place. I suspect that his desk at the National Institutes of Allergy and Infectious Diseases is surrounded by eggshells. I believe that even though my newspaper went out of business in 1997, *New York Native* remains a thorn in his psyche to this very day. I doubt that he can hear the words "Chronic Fatigue Syndrome," "HHV-6," or "Peter Duesberg" without thinking of *New York Native.*

Two of my reporters paid a price for their association with *New York Native.* He was dramatically rude to one reporter when she showed up on the same TV show with him. He refused to shake the hand of another reporter when he was introduced to him at a medical conference. Not surprising since I have already pointed out in the chapter above that Fauci basically said that members of the media would lose precious access if they didn't play ball.

I will give credit to Fauci for being astute in recognizing my newspaper as his bête noire because it does contain all the journalistic ingredients necessary for his eventual downfall. In my book about *New York Native, The Chronic Fatigue Syndrome Epidemic Cover-up,* you can watch the evolution of the Fauci Ponzi scheme from the beginning of the AIDS epidemic into the early years of the deftly handled Chronic Fatigue Syndrome cover-up.

From my experience covering the CDC and Fauci's antics I now believe that scientific totalitarianism is fertile ground for medical and scientific Ponzi schemes. And when you find scientific Ponzi schemes, you know you have also encountered a culture of scientific totalitarianism. From watching Fauci and his public health puppets closely, I have constructed a list of the elements necessary for a successful public health Ponzi scheme.

1. Nosological fraud. (That's the branch of medicine dealing with the classification of disease. It is ground zero for public health fraud.)

2. Epidemiological fraud.

3. Virological fraud.

4. Treatment fraud. (Treatments that harm more than they heal or conceal more than they reveal.)

5. Public health policy fraud.

6. Concealment of negative scientific data and paradigm-challenging anomalies.

7. Use of an elite network of "old boys" and pseudo-activist provocateurs to censor critics and whistleblowers.

8. Chronic obscurantism.

9. If necessary, vigilantism and witch-hunts against any intellectuals, scientists, or citizens who constitute any form of resistance to the Ponzi scheme.

10. A subservient scientific press that is used as a conveyor belt for the Ponzi scheme's propaganda.

While you could say that it took a village to put these elements into place, there really is only one person who has been able to control all the aspects of the Ponzi scheme the way Leonard Bernstein controlled an orchestra. Anthony Fauci has been richly rewarded for his ability to keep this Ponzi scheme going, just as Bernie Madoff was for his. These are just some of the awards Fauci received:

1979: Arthur S. Flemming Award

1990: International Chiron Award for Biomedical Research and Training, from Accademia Nazionale di Medicina - Italy

1995: Ernst Jung Prize (shared with Samuel A. Wells, Jr.)[9]

2002: Albany Medical Center Prize

2005: National Medal of Science

2005: American Association of Immunologists Lifetime Achievement Award

2007: Mary Woodard Lasker Public Service Award

2008: Presidential Medal of Freedom

2013: Robert Koch Gold Medal

2013: Prince Mahidol Award

2016: John Dirks Canada Gairdner Global Health Award

Fauci is one of the highest paid people in the government. I leave it to historians to sort out how much he made from his scientific Ponzi scheme. Journalist Terry Michael was working on a book about Fauci's ill-gotten gains but, unfortunately, died before he could finish it.

If you search Google for articles or blogs that are critical of Fauci, except for a few notable examples (my work and Hillary Johnson's) you will come up empty handed.

Journalism about Fauci tends to be uninformed, uncritical, and lionizing. The most iconic piece about him was the canonization he received from a nun. In a Catholic News Agency article, Sister Joan L. Roccasalvo wrote, "Dr. Fauci is blessed with a first-class temperament crowning his other achievements. This, despite his own admission of being a perfectionist. Some years ago, at the height of the AIDS controversy, I listened to him delivering a lecture. In the Q&A, one person after the other lashed out at him. Quick to size up, deliberate to respond, this preppy-looking physician answered calmly and without condescension. His style: cool. Later he observed that the audience was lashing out at everyone and not at him in particular. He had walked with them in their pain. He absorbed their pain. Wasn't this Christ's way? And what of St. Luke, the physician, whose gospel is permeated with compassion for the most vulnerable?"

Sister Joan L. Roccasalvo outdid herself when she ended her piece by noting " . . . Dr. Fauci's inspiration cannot be measured. In fact, the beauty of such a life is the surest and most persuasive occasion to form disciples of the Lord and build a better world. God's love shines out from those who, of themselves, are unaware of God's limitless power working in their lives for good. So it is with Anthony Fauci, a man for others, a universal treasure."

To that, one can only say what must be uttered when he speaks at NIH: "Amen." Fauci knew the importance of good public relations. He could have taught Bernie Madoff a thing or two about working a crowd. If the nuns are on your side you have nothing to worry about. See if you can find a You

Tube moment when Rachel Maddow tells Fauci that she thinks he is "a great American."

When Madoff's Ponzi scheme was eventually exposed, it was shocking how obvious the scam was. Boston financial analyst Harry Markopolos, the man who figured out what Madoff was up to, told *60 Minutes*, "It took me five minutes to know that it was a fraud. It took me another almost four hours of mathematical modeling to prove it was a fraud." There was no shortage of people who discerned the glaring irregularities in the "science" that bolstered Fauci's Ponzi scheme. In addition to the reporters at *New York Native*, there was a fascinating group of scientists and intellectuals I discuss in *Peter Duesberg and the Duesbergians*.

In some ways, you could say that Fauci's Ponzi scheme has survived for so long because his critics were too nice. Assuming that norms were being maintained, they were often collegial, hoping that reason would prevail. It would not. It's a shame that Fauci's critics didn't recognize that they were really whistleblowers and scientific crime-fighters. They would politely make their points in a Fauci universe where critics were welcome to get jobs at Starbucks. You can't reason with someone who has Fauci's power and administrative long arms because at all times he is running and protecting a criminal enterprise. His fake science is always covertly fighting for its life.

Two communities especially have failed to grasp the nature of Fauci's HIV Ponzi scheme and paid a terrible price for it: the gay community and the Chronic Fatigue Syndrome community. The gay community and the Chronic Fatigue Syndrome community are now victims of a massive epidemic associated with the HHV-6/7/8 family of viruses. I will have more to say about this in a future book, but anyone who wants to explore the implications of the HHV-6/7/8 epidemic should check out the over 3,000 posts on my website, HHV-6 University.

It's very sad that the Chronic Fatigue Syndrome community has never challenged the HIV/AIDS pseudoscience of Anthony Fauci. While there is a great deal of CFS-related hostility toward Fauci, it generally revolves around *neglect* of Chronic Fatigue Syndrome rather than the *cover-up* of the obvious fact that what has been called AIDS and what has been called Chronic Fatigue Syndrome are really just two different faces of one epidemic driven by the HHV-6/7/8 family of viruses.

When new retroviruses were found in Chronic Fatigue Syndrome patients by scientists Elaine DeFreitas and Judy Mikovits, the work was not discredited just because the retroviruses would show that CFS is real. The truth is that it was undermined because the work threatened to show that Chronic Fatigue Syndrome is just another iteration of the AIDS epidemic. Judy Mikovits, the scientist whose work on XMRV, a mouse retrovirus she claimed to find in CFS patients, was initially the object of international adulation from CFS community. But a scientist connected with the AIDS establishment pulled the rug out from under her work by "de-discovering XMRV," to the great disappointment to CFS patients and activists. If the CFS community knew the truth about AIDS and Fauci's Ponzi scheme, they could have turned the tables on scientists who sent Mikovits into exile because of her retroviral findings. They never asked whether HIV could have been "de-discovered" as the cause of AIDS if it had been as critically vetted as XMRV. I believe that one day historians will conclude that finding a retrovirus in CFS patients would have sent scientists quickly down a slippery slope to an understanding that *HIV is not the real cause of AIDS and AIDS is not HIV disease.* What has been called "AIDS" is on a spectrum of illness caused by the HHV-6/7/8 family of viruses. And that would not be a good development for Anthony Fauci's brilliant Ponzi scheme.

Because Fauci is close to retirement, he may never have to answer for the crisis he has created. I have spent more than half of my life covering his scientific Ponzi scheme. I am hopeful that these books (below) that I have written since the demise of *New York Native* will help future generations clean up the biomedical, political, and cultural mess left by the Fauci Ponzi scheme.

The Chronic Fatigue Syndrome Epidemic Cover-up: How a Little Newspaper Solved the Biggest Scientific and Political Mystery of Our Time

The Chronic Fatigue Syndrome Epidemic Cover-up Volume Two: The Origins of Totalitarianism in Science and Medicine

Peter Duesberg and the Duesbergians: How a Brave and Brilliant Group of Scientists Challenged the AIDS Establishment and Inadvertently Exposed the Chronic Fatigue Syndrome Epidemic

The Closing Argument: A shocking courtroom novella about AIDS, Chronic Fatigue Syndrome, racial injustice and HHV-6, the virus that threatens us all

The Stonewall Massacre

The African Swine Fever Novel

The Black Party: A Dramatic Comedy in Two Acts

The Last Lovers on Earth: Stories from Dark Times

Iron Peter: A Year in the Mythopoetic Life of New York City

Butterfly Ghosts and The New Hippocratic Oath: Earlier and Later Poems

Made in the USA
Coppell, TX
05 May 2020

24480485R00030